YOUR MOUTH— YOUR LIFE

The Connection of Oral Health To Whole Body Health

By Jean–Max Jean–Pierre, D.D.S., M.D.S.

ACKNOWLEDGEMENT

This book is dedicated to my family, my wife Daisy and the girls, Gigi and Demi. Thank you for your love and support. To my PCC team, thank you for being part of the vision in helping to bring health to the nations; you are all 10's. Special thanks to Deborah Bush for editing my manuscript. Thank you to Dr. Bradley Bale for your encouragement, I am grateful.

Dr. Jean-Pierre has provided a wonderful and informative discussion regarding the importance of oral health to total health and wellness. "Your Mouth Your Life" is unique in its simple and easy to understand approach using examples that emphasize the concepts of healthy lifestyle choices and the benefits they bring to achieving a balanced and satisfying existence. The stress and distractions of daily life make it all too easy to neglect ourselves; however, we must make the commitment to maintaining optimal oral health in order to achieve whole body wellness. The relationship between oral inflammation and chronic systemic inflammatory diseases/conditions such as cardiovascular disease, diabetes, arthritis, respiratory disease, and dementia cannot be ignored. Individuals with optimal oral health will experience reduced morbidity and mortality from systemic inflammatory burden as they age. Dr. Jean-Pierre is among the young dynamic leaders within the health professions and his book demonstrates his ability to blend current scientific information with superb clinical skills to improve the quality of life for his patients and the public.

Anthony M. Iacopino DMD PhD
Dean, College of Dentistry
Executive Director, International Centre for Oral-Systemic Health
Professor, Dental Diagnostic and Surgical Sciences
University of Manitoba - Rady Faculty of Health Sciences

"Dr. Jean-Max Jean-Pierre has done what others in the dental profession have been challenged to do. He has provided the general public and the medical profession at large, with a timely and relevant guidebook of sorts, based on the most current scientific research relating to the mouth/body connection.

Your Mouth – Your Life is an easy to read summation of the significant connections between - and even life-threatening consequences of -

oral disease and disease in the rest of the body. Dr. Jean-Pierre has clearly and succinctly spelled out the critical importance of improved oral health and its relationship to total body wellness, while offering sound advice and leading-edge treatment modalities as options for BEST health."

Dr. Lisa Marie Samaha, DDS, FAGD
Founder and Lead Instructor, Perio Arts Institute
"Transforming the Way Dental Practices Heal their Patients"

"Whole – body Health: the new paradigm in health care delivery. This crucial concept is promoted by the National Institutes of Health (NIH), Centers for Disease Control (CDC), and all health organizations. While the concept itself is not new, the clinical trials that support this model are. In fact, medical research in every important arena supports the role of all health professionals working together to make this concept possible. Clinical trials also explain why "Oral Health and Oral Medicine" must be included in order to achieve "Whole – Body Health".

Preventing Type 2 Diabetes, heart disease and strokes cannot be achieved without achieving Optimal Oral Health and this cannot be achieved without achieving Optimal Periodontal Health.

Clinicians from every medical discipline must recognize these advances that connect the dots between the risks associated with Oral Diseases, especially periodontal diseases, and their relevance to the morbidity and mortality of every chronic disease.

"Your Mouth – Your Life" is an excellent resource for aiding clinicians and patients that want to undertake their own responsibility of achieving their own "Whole – Body Health".

Thomas W. Nabors, DDS, FACD
Adjunct Professor University of Tennessee Health Science Center (UTHSC)
Founder Oral DNA Labs
Chief Dental Officer, Quest Diagnostics (Retired)

Dr. Jean-Pierre concisely illustrates why you get better health and longevity as you heed this easy-to-read brief expert's view. With his guidance, you will see that effective mouth care may not be exactly what you thought. You are free to think a bit further, how you will benefit in your life that your money is going to be spent more likely on what you want instead of repairs and damage control all over your body—your body that serves you better and allows you to do what you want more and longer.

John A. Stewart, MD
Board Certified Anatomic and Clinical Pathology
Board Certified Family Medicine

TABLE OF CONTENTS

FOREWORD

By Bradley F. Bale, M.D.

Our bodies have approximately 60,000 miles of arteries and veins. These channels unite every aspect of us. We are constantly bathed throughout these channels by the same blood. It is fantasy to believe one part of the body exists in total isolation from another part. The gum tissue in our mouth is heavily enriched with vessels. The many germs found in our oral cavity can get into these channels and then take a trip to any part of our bodies. The extensive vascular highway allows your mouth to communicate with your entire body.

Medicine and dentistry conceptually have been separated by an imaginary boundary. People think they see a dentist to just take care of what is in their mouth. People believe they need to see a medical doctor to take care of all the other parts of the body. What the public needs to understand is that keeping the mouth healthy contributes to their general wellness. A sick mouth can make the whole body ill. Dentistry is a vital component of medical care.

One very important area in which oral health is intertwined with systemic health involves the arterial highway. Diseased arteries are responsible for virtually all heart attacks and the vast majority of strokes. Heart attacks are still the number one killer in this country. Every thirty-four seconds someone suffers a heart attack, and every minute someone dies from one. Sudden cardiac death is responsible for the greatest burden of years of productive life lost. It is estimated that men lose two million years and women 1.3 million years of productive life annually due to death from coronary artery disease. Every forty seconds, someone suffers a stroke, and every four minutes, someone dies from a stroke.

There is unequivocal evidence that diseased gums are independently associated with diseased arteries. Heart attack and stroke risk are increased when the gums are infected with certain harmful germs. Recent evidence indicates abscessed teeth may trigger a lot of heart attacks. The care your dental professional delivers impacts your chance of developing arterial disease, which will impact your risk of heart attack and stroke.

We live in an exciting era of technology and science. Dentistry can now accurately determine through DNA testing the presence of specific harmful bacteria and their concentration. Studies are available indicating it is the burden of certain bacteria in the mouth that drives the arterial risk. Examination of the mouth is still important for the depth of gum pockets, attachment loss of teeth, and presence of bleeding gums, but these somewhat subjective measurements are now greatly enhanced by sophisticated lab testing. In addition, dentists are now able to take 3D images of the teeth that can illustrate previously invisible abscesses. These dental tests will greatly enhance overall health. Dentistry currently exists in a marvelous time of technical laboratory tests and knowledge.

All of the above is not only superb for our well being, but it also is financially beneficial. Recent research has shown that the dollars spent on maintaining a healthy mouth return dividends worth many times what the initial investment cost. This was not only shown for reduced expenditures for heart attacks and strokes, but also for reduced medical care in diabetics. The old saying, "put your money where your mouth is," should take on a whole new meaning!

The material you are about to read was written by a leader in the oral-systemic field of healthcare. Dr. Jean-Max Jean-Pierre, D.D.S., M.D.S. possesses an in-depth understanding of the critical importance of sustaining a healthy mouth in order to have overall wellness. Read carefully his words of wisdom. Words from his mouth can save your life.

Dr. Bradley F. Bale is one of the nation's leading specialists in preventing heart attacks, stroke and diabetes. Since 2001, he has given numerous presentations to medical and dental groups in the US and abroad.

Convinced that standard of care wasn't doing enough to identify early stages of CVD and avert recurrences in heart attack and stroke survivors, he cofounded the Bale/Doneen Method with Amy Doneen in 2001. Four years ago this personalized approach of CV risk assessment and management evolved to an effectiveness level sufficient enough to allow them to attach a 'guarantee' to their clinical practices.

Their research on CVD prevention has been published in such respected medical journals as Atherosclerosis, Post Graduate Medicine, Journal of the National Medical Association, Journal of Clinical Lipidology, Physician's Weekly, Alternative Therapies in Health and Medicine and ADVANCE for Healthy Aging. Dr. Bale has also served as a reviewer for American Journal of Cardiology, International Journal of Clinical and Experimental Cardiology, Archives of Medical Science, Journal of Cardiovascular Nursing and the CDC's Preventing Chronic Disease. He is the co-author with Amy Doleen of the 2014 book BEAT THE HEART ATTACK GENE (Wiley General Trade, New York, NY). He was a keynote speaker at the 4th International Conference on Clinical & Experimental Cardiology April 14, 2014 in San Antonio, TX.

INTRODUCTION

I have always believed that each of us has a purpose—a role to play that allows us to impact the world in a positive way. I also believe that God often places in our hearts certain desires that lead us to fulfill this purpose. My goals and desires have led me to become an advocate for good oral health as a means of heightening awareness about systemic health. As you read this story, I hope you will see why.

I was eight years old when my mother moved from our native Haiti to the United States. My younger sister had heart disease, and the most effective treatment was offered in Chicago. After my sister's condition had stabilized, my mother decided to stay in America, with the hope of one day bringing the rest of us over. It would be five long years before we were finally able to join her in the States. It was a dream come true.

We moved to Florida, attended school, and gradually began to understand the vast opportunities that exist in the US. My mother and stepfather had always emphasized the importance of education, and over time, they began to notice my interest in healthcare. One day, my stepfather suggested that I look into dentistry, and because I greatly respected his opinion, I decided to explore this path. The more I researched, the more fascinated I became. By the time I was in high school, I was telling my teachers, and anyone else who would listen, that I was going to be a dentist.

That's not to say there weren't some bumps along the road. While at the University of South Florida, I attended a meeting of the pre-dental society. The first time I saw a local dentist showing slides of a surgical procedure, I became so queasy that I had to excuse myself from the room. Yet, twenty years later, here I am, passionate about restoring people to health by performing periodontal surgery.

My family also went through trials that deeply affected me on a personal and professional level. One of my younger brothers was a very talented football player; some even said he could go professional one day. I remember like it was yesterday when I received a call that he had fainted at football practice. He was later diagnosed with cardiomyopathy, or an enlargement of the heart muscle, and he had to be taken to the University of Florida in Gainesville for treatment. Unfortunately, that condition prevented him from becoming a professional football player. Today, he has a fulfilling career as a college counselor, helping students find the right career path. My older sister would later experience heart problems as well.

My siblings' health crises motivated me to help others desire and achieve health, not only when it comes to their mouths, but in a holistic sense. Throughout my career as a periodontal specialist, I have followed the growing body of research linking periodontal disease with other systemic conditions. Moreover, I regularly see this link in my practice. I have diagnosed many forms of periodontal disease in patients ranging from seven to ninety years of age. Several of these patients have subsequently been diagnosed with a systemic disease, among these include hypertension, diabetes, rheumatoid arthritis, osteoporosis and oral cancer.

The "case studies" that follow in this publication are stories about patients in my practice. Their stories will open your eyes to the realities of periodontal disease and how it affects the individual's overall health.

The American Heart Association has stated that heart disease is a silent killer, but I believe periodontal disease is an excellent tool to help medical professionals discover cardiovascular issues before they advance to a critical stage. The focus of my work is to educate people about how they can use periodontal assessments and treatment to gauge and improve the state of their overall health, in addition to their oral health.

CHAPTER 1

THE MOUTH–BODY CONNECTION

People are more health–conscious today than at any other point in history. We understand the connection between our life choices and the condition of our bodies; we also know that our mental and spiritual health has a profound effect on our health. We are no longer satisfied with compartmentalizing our heath concerns—now, *holistic health* is the goal. Yet despite this, many of us continue to think of oral health as somehow separate from the rest of the body. You have a toothache, you go to the dentist, he or she administers treatment, and that's the end of the story. But the truth is that what is going on in your mouth is interrelated with and often indicative of your overall well being.

Gum disease (including gingivitis and periodontitis), which will be described in this publication, is pervasive throughout the United States. In fact, the Centers for Disease Control and Prevention (CDC) reported in 2012 that gum disease affects almost 50% of the American population (47.2%). This means 64.7 million Americans over the age of 30 have gum diseases. Severe periodontal (gum) disease, called "periodontitis," is found in 15–20% of middle–aged (35–44 years) adults and may result in tooth loss. Globally, about 30% of people aged 65–74 have no natural teeth.

The common symptoms are:

Bleeding gums when brushing or flossing

- Tender, red or swollen gums
- Gums pulling away from the teeth
- Bad breath, even after brushing
- Pain when chewing food
- Loose teeth

Gum disease is the result of inflammation. One of the key messages of this publication is that inflammation of the mouth is linked to systemic (whole body) inflammation, and the consequences of not treating the inflammation can be grave. Men, beware. Gum disease affects 56.4% of all American men. Women, 38.4% of you are affected—more than one in three. If you are a smoker, you have a higher risk with 64.2% battling the disease. The word battling is not used loosely, since treating the disease and eliminating its causes to prevent future occurrences can be quite difficult.

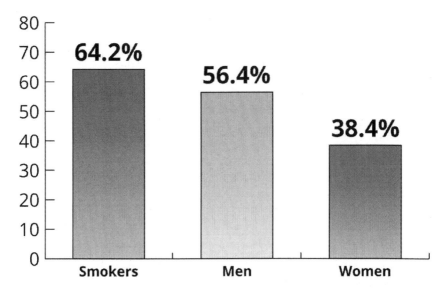

Here's why you should care. Not only does untreated gum disease lead to tooth, bone and soft tissue infection in the mouth and often tooth loss; it also affects your overall health and can shorten your life.

Established and emerging science continues to link chronic low-grade infection in the mouth with inflammation that impacts all systems of the body.

The relationship between oral diseases and systemic disease has been heavily researched over the years, with the bulk of the literature focused on the roles that inflammation and bacteria play in the mouth–body connection. Bacteria in the mouth not only contributes to cavities and oral cancer, it can also be transferred to the lungs, create rheumatoid arthritis in the jaw joints, and cause chronic headaches. It can exacerbate and be a contributing factor to all inflammatory diseases of the body, for example, diabetes, cardiovascular/cerebrovascular disease, kidney disease, respiratory disease, arthritis, osteoporosis, dementia, obesity, metabolic syndrome, inflammatory bowel disease, and cancer. It can even be a contributor to adverse pregnancy outcomes. Untreated inflammation in the mouth elevates levels of systemic inflammation and may actually cause vascular disease, respiratory disease, dementia, and diabetes in otherwise healthy individuals.

Since periodontal disease is recognized as a medical problem, physicians have a responsibility to consider chronic oral infections as a possible reason for, or warning sign of, systemic inflammation. Today, progressive dentists and physicians are collaborating on patient care. They understand that the significance of numerous mouth–body connections cannot be overestimated.

If you want to lead the healthiest, longest life you can, you must take into account the importance of preventing and treating oral disease. When you are aware of the risks, causes and symptoms of periodontal disease, and the connection between oral health and other health issues, you will want to take an active role in your own oral healthcare.

Your Mouth—Gateway to Your Body

Your mouth is obviously the port of entry for food nutrients entering your body. The foods you eat influence the nutritional status of your body and in turn your health. Strong research based evidence indicates poor oral health is a silent factor with high potential to promote systemic diseases. According to the American Dental Association, poor oral health leads to degenerative diseases that contribute to millions of deaths in the United States each year.

The phrase "you are what you eat" applies to dental health as well as systemic health. The food we eat impacts the health of our teeth and gums.

Research reveals that consuming sugary foods and carbonated beverages destroys tooth enamel, as well as increases the risk of gum diseases. In fact, the negative effects are directly correlated with the degree of food refinement. Conversely, poor oral health can impact food choices and nutritional status.[1] For example, tooth sensitivity and bleeding gums are often the reasons why people avoid certain foods that are rich in nutrients. The discomfort associated with food motivates them to reach out for more processed convenience foods such as sugary nutritional shakes.

Studies link diets high in convenience foods with inflammation inside the body.[2,3] Inflammation is among the top 5 reasons for many degenerative diseases like heart disease, stroke, diabetes, including neuro degenerative diseases like Alzheimer's. Changing the diet to fresh, whole foods reduces inflammation.

Inflammation

We have all experienced inflammation at one point or another—that uncomfortable swelling, pain and redness. It may be from a bug bite, a bump on the head, or even a virus. As unpleasant as it is, inflammation is actually a critical function of our immune system. When we are injured or come into contact with a virus or bacteria, the white blood cells rush to the site to protect our bodies from further harm. The result is inflammation. When the inflammation is unchecked or chronic, it can damage tissues and bones, sometimes leading to tooth loss. Moreover, chronic inflammation can lead to dangerous and even life-threatening conditions such as heart disease, diabetes, rheumatoid arthritis, autoimmune diseases, and even Alzheimer's disease. Recent studies have concluded that inflammation is a hallmark response to bacteria or bacteria in the bloodstream and that inflammation is not only linked to both oral and systemic diseases, but is also a link between oral and systemic diseases.[4,5,6]

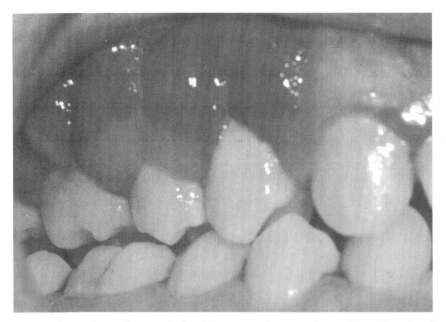

Research confirms that periodontitis—gum disease—is not just a localized infection but also is indicative of inflammatory illness elsewhere in the body.

Our mouths are teeming with bacteria. Think of all the things you might touch in a day that may be contaminated (money is a great example); now imagine touching them, and then popping a piece of gum into your mouth. It's that easy. When the gums and teeth are compromised, the bacteria in your mouth, as well as viruses, gain entry into the bloodstream, travelling it like a highway to other systems of the body. That is why it is so critical to go for regular periodontal assessments and receive treatment as needed.

Overall Health

Many people believe that if they get through cold and flu season without getting sick, they are healthy; but the truth is, true health is much more than the absence of illness. It is the presence of balance among the various systems of the body. Achieving this balance takes commitment to exercise, eating nutritious foods, getting enough rest, and seeking the appropriate healthcare—all preventive and to treat disease.

We are all born with a different genetic makeup—the heart disease in my family, for example. We all face different health challenges. There is also a growing acceptance—even within the traditional medical community, that our mental and spiritual states have an effect upon our physical well being.

Nutrition

As I stated above, the purpose of this book is to educate people about the role our oral health plays in our overall health. One of the biggest factors in maintaining a healthy mouth is nutrition. But what, you might ask, are the best foods to eat for optimal health? It seems that every day there is another diet, another list of foods that one should or should not consume. Again, the answer is balance.

Barring any medical conditions that carry specific restrictions, most healthcare providers recommend a diet rich in fruits, vegetables, whole grains and complex carbohydrates—sweet potatoes, not French fries! It is also important to get enough protein, with fish and chicken being the best options. Red meat is fine in moderation; and we should keep salt, fats, and sugars to a minimum.

When it comes to oral health, sugar is clearly the greatest threat. People typically consume the most sugary snacks between meals. No matter what you have done in the past, you can decide to make a different choice moving forward. Munch on vegetables, fruits, low fat cheese and nuts.

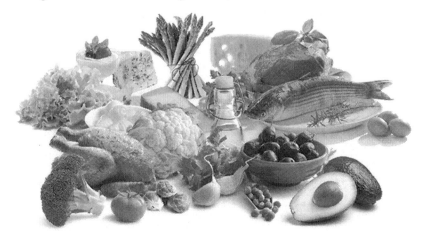

CHAPTER 2

PERIODONTAL DISEASE

Your teeth are supported by gums and bones. When inflammation occurs in these areas, it is called **periodontal disease**. According to CDC reports, nearly half of the United States population suffers from some form of periodontal disease. The condition can range from mild gum inflammation to severe inflammatory conditions that eventually lead to tooth loss.

If the inflammation is only on the outer surface of the gums, it is called **gingivitis**. If the inflammation occurs in the connecting tissue and bone, it is called **periodontitis**. People who want to preserve their teeth for their lifetime should seek the regular care of a dentist or dental specialist to control the bacteria that cause periodontal inflammation and to treat any inflammation in its mildest to advancing forms. The consequences of untreated gum inflammation can be grave.

Normal tooth

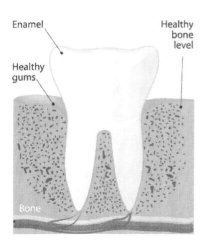

Enamel

Healthy bone level

Healthy gums

Bone

Periodontitis

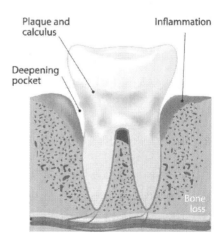

Plaque and calculus

Inflammation

Deepening pocket

Bone loss

Gingivitis

Gingivitis is the mildest form of periodontal disease. It causes the gums to become red, swollen, and bleed easily. There is usually little or no discomfort at this stage, and many people do not recognize they have it. Gingivitis is often caused by inadequate oral hygiene. Gingivitis is reversible with professional treatment and good oral home care.

Factors that may contribute to gingivitis include diabetes, smoking, aging, genetic predisposition, systemic diseases and conditions, stress, inadequate nutrition, puberty, hormonal fluctuations, pregnancy, substance abuse, HIV infection, and certain medication use.

Periodontitis

Untreated gingivitis can advance to periodontitis. With time, colonizing bacteria that create the biofilm called **plaque** can spread and grow below the gum line. Toxins produced by the bacteria in plaque irritate the gums. The toxins stimulate a chronic inflammatory response in which the body turns on itself, and the tissues and bone that support the teeth are broken down and destroyed. The gum tissue then separates from the teeth, forming pockets (spaces between the teeth and gums) that become infected. As the disease progresses, the pockets deepen and more gum tissue and bone are destroyed. Often, this destructive process has very mild symptoms at the start—but as it advances, teeth can become loose and may have to be removed.

There are many forms of periodontitis. The most common ones include the following:

- **Aggressive periodontitis** occurs in patients who are otherwise clinically healthy. Common features include rapid attachment loss, bone destruction, and multiple occurrence of the condition within families, either due to genetics or environmental similarities.

- **Chronic periodontitis** results in inflammation within the supporting tissues of the teeth, progressive attachment and bone loss. This is the most frequently occurring form of periodontitis and is characterized by pocket formation and/or recession of the gingiva. It is prevalent in adults, although it can occur at any age. Progression of attachment loss usually occurs slowly, but periods of rapid progression can occur.

- **Periodontitis as a manifestation of systemic diseases** often begins at a young age. Systemic conditions such as heart disease, respiratory disease, and diabetes are associated with this form of periodontitis.

- **Necrotizing periodontal disease** is an infection characterized by the localized death of gingival tissues, periodontal ligament and alveolar bone. These lesions are most commonly observed in individuals with systemic conditions such as HIV infection, malnutrition and immunosuppression.

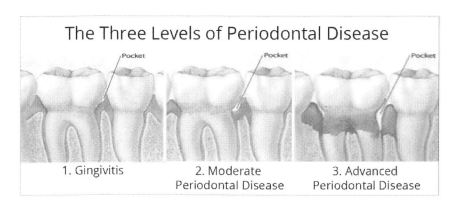

The Three Levels of Periodontal Disease

1. Gingivitis   2. Moderate Periodontal Disease   3. Advanced Periodontal Disease

Risk Factors for Periodontal Disease

Did you know that pregnant women and people with crooked teeth are at a greater risk for gum disease? There are many risks for gum disease. Some, like smoking or chewing tobacco, are well known. While others, like oral contraceptives and chemotherapy, may surprise you.

Those with a family history of poor oral health are at greater risk for periodontitis, as are people with compromised immune systems (e.g. those living with HIV/AIDS). As mentioned earlier, there is also a strong link between periodontitis and diabetes; therefore, people with type 2 diabetes should be especially diligent in getting assessments of their oral health and early treatment.

Researchers point out that we need to be aware of the following risk factors for periodontal diseases:

- **Smoking:** Among the many health impacts of smoking, gum disease is a significant one.

- **Diabetes:** If you have chronic high blood sugar or diabetes your immune system may not function efficiently. If your immune system does not fight bad bacteria in your mouth effectively, it forms the sticky biofilm called plaque that grows below the gum line.

- **Certain medications:** Over a period of time, certain medications can reduce the secretion of saliva and can give you dry mouth. Dry mouth increases the susceptibility for gum disease.

- **Genetic factors:** If you have a close family member with a history of periodontal disease, you have a higher risk.

- **Poor dental hygiene:** If you do not brush daily or floss periodically, you may be more susceptible to gum disease. The good news is that milder forms of gum disease can be reversed by proper oral hygiene and regular visits to your dentist.

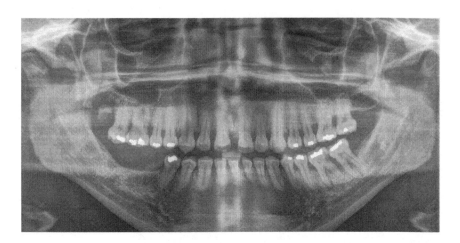

Diagnosis of Periodontal Disease

Before treatment begins, your oral health will be evaluated. The evaluation includes questions about your medical and dental history, a dental exam, and radiographs. Factors that could affect the disease or treatment will be reviewed. For example, if you have had a heart valve or joint replacement, you may need to take antibiotics before some or all of your dental treatments.

Your dental history will be evaluated. Your cleaning and periodontal treatment history will be reviewed. You will be asked about past dental work such as crowns, bridges, and dental implants. You will be asked about any dental work you plan to have done. There will be conversation about how you've been taking care of your teeth and ways you can improve home care.

During your exam, your gums will be checked for bleeding, firmness, recession, and sensitivity. You will be examined for signs of gradual tooth movement and movement that occurs with direct pressure. You will be examined for bite problems that could affect periodontal disease and its treatment. If a medical problem such as diabetes or heart disease is a factor, you'll be referred to your medical doctor. Radiographs that show each tooth, including the roots and surrounding bone, will be taken. This helps detect bone loss.

One way to check for gum damage and bone loss is to measure how deep the pockets are between the gum tissue and your teeth. A special periodontal instrument is used, and the depths are recorded in your patient record. A healthy depth is 1 to 3 millimeters. Pockets deeper than 3 indicate your delicate periodontal tissue is at risk. The deeper the pocket is, the greater the inflammation present.

After your evaluation, your treatment options will be discussed. In many cases, non-surgical treatments are performed first. This may be the only treatment needed, or it may be the first step in preparing for surgery or laser periodontal therapy. In some cases, surgery or laser periodontal therapy is planned from the onset. Following any planned treatment, ongoing professional hygiene maintenance (teeth cleaning in the dental office) is needed to keep the disease under control.

Depending on the extent or severity of your gum infection, saliva DNA testing may be recommended. This type of testing can identify and measures certain bacteria in your mouth that cause gingivitis and periodontal disease, determine if you are more likely to develop more serious gum disease, and determine if you are at increased risk for HPV–related oral and throat cancers.

Treatment for Periodontal Disease

Like any other medical problems, the course of treatment for gum disease will depend on the severity of the condition. There are many treatment options for periodontal disease. Gingivitis is reversible with professional treatment and good oral hygiene. In its early stages, a dental professional can treat it without surgery. He or she will prescribe an antibiotic mouthwash or other medication, or if necessary, perform a deep scaling (cleaning below the gum line) or root planing (which removes diseased parts of the tooth). Sometimes all that is needed is a thorough teeth cleaning. Just remember to make regular cleaning appointments.

The American Academy of Periodontology (AAP) shares a summary description of various treatment procedures with the Public on it's website (www.perio.org).

Non–Surgical Treatment

The goal of non–surgical treatment is to create conditions that enable tissues in the mouth to heal. This is done by reducing plaque, infection, and other causes of periodontal disease. Standard non–surgical treatment is **scaling** (deep cleaning below the gum line) and **root planing** (removing diseased parts of the tooth below the gum line). An ultrasonic tool may be used, and antibiotics may be given. Limited research suggests that laser treatment as an adjunct to scaling and root planing may be beneficial; therefore, laser therapy may be included. A re–evaluation is performed in about 4–8 weeks following treatment to check the periodontal status. Additional treatment may be required, depending on the conclusion of the re–evaluation.

Bite Correction

Bite correction may be recommended if your periodontal health is being affected by a poor bite that makes it difficult to fully brush and floss your teeth, or a bite that places excessive pressure on your teeth due to the way your teeth meet when you bite, chew, and grind your teeth against each other. Orthodontics can properly align your teeth, and modification of the tops of the teeth can help equalize the forces on them when your teeth come together. Bite correction will increase the ability to maintain gingival health after appropriate treatment of the inflammation.

Surgical Treatments

Patients who have suffered the ravages of periodontal disease are commonly in need of full mouth rehabilitation. The patient's dentist works with an interdisciplinary team of specialists as needed. Among those specialists are periodontists.

Periodontists are dentistry's experts in treating periodontal disease and performing periodontal surgical procedures. They receive up to three additional years of specialized training in periodontal disease treatment—both surgical and non-surgical treatments, periodontal plastic surgery procedures, and replacing missing teeth with dental implants.

In order to further increase surgical effectiveness, minimally invasive periodontal surgery (MIPS) includes the use of operating microscopes with microsurgical instruments and lasers. Lasers may be used in surgical periodontal treatment, and when used properly by expert clinicians, there is less bleeding, swelling, and discomfort to the patient.

Periodontists are exceptionally well trained and skilled in performing the following surgical treatments. Your comfort and post-operative care will be given careful attention.

- **Pocket Reduction:** Your bone and gum tissue should fit snugly around your teeth like a turtleneck around your neck. When you have periodontal disease, this supporting tissue and bone are destroyed, forming "pockets" around the teeth. Over time, these pockets become deeper, providing a larger space for bacteria to live. As bacteria develop around the teeth, they can accumulate and advance under the gum tissue. These deep pockets collect even more bacteria, resulting in further bone and tissue loss. Eventually, if too much bone is lost, the teeth will need to be extracted. If you have deep gum pockets, the gum tissue can be folded back, and disease-causing bacteria can be removed before securing the gum tissue back in place. Any irregular surfaces of the damaged bone can be smoothed to limit areas where disease-causing bacteria can hide. This procedure allows the gum tissue to better reattach to healthy bone and is used when simple scaling and root planning have been ineffective.

- **Gum Graft Surgery:** When the gum has receded beyond the crown and the root is exposed, it is often desirable to re-cover the root surface. This is primarily done for cosmetic reasons, but it is also advisable if there is root sensitivity. There may also be a lack of attached (hard) gum tissue, and the root coverage surgery is designed to correct that problem at the same time. Gum grafts can be surgically placed to cover roots or develop gum tissue at the sites where gum tissue has receded. The periodontist will use gum tissue taken from the palate of your mouth or another donor source in order to cover the exposed root. This can be done for one tooth or several teeth to protect tooth roots, reduce sensitivity, and cosmetically shape your gum line into naturally aesthetic contours. (See Figure A)

- **Bone Regeneration:** If bone supporting your teeth has been destroyed by periodontal disease, a bone regenerative procedure may be recommended. The periodontist will fold back the gum tissue and remove disease–causing bacteria. Membranes (filters), bone grafts or tissue–stimulating proteins can be surgically placed to encourage your body's natural ability to regenerate lost bone tissue. This MIPS technique also allows for minimization of soft tissue trauma and the removal of granulation tissue from periodontal defects using a much smaller surgical incision than typically used in standard bone graft techniques. Even if you opt to replace a missing tooth or teeth with a traditional dental bridge instead of an implant restoration, bone regeneration may be recommended if periodontal disease has left indentations in the gums and jawbone.

Note: Bone Regeneration is also called "Ridge Augmentation." The alveolar ridge of the jaw is the bone that surrounds the roots of teeth. Sometimes, when a tooth is lost or removed, the empty bone socket is left to heal on its own. Many clinicians now fill an empty socket with osseous material after extracting a tooth in order to help preserve the previous height and width of the ridge. If an empty socket is not filled by a clinician and does not fill with bone on its own, the surrounding bone can break (cave in around the socket). Not only does this leave insufficient bone for a dental implant but this also creates an unaesthetic effect when replacing the missing tooth with a bridge or denture. Many times, bone degeneration continues to occur, affecting the facial features as well as the smile. Bone regeneration (described above) is the procedure used to rebuild the bone of the alveolar ridge and restore it to a height and width suitable for dental implant placement or for aesthetic purposes.

- **Tooth Extraction:** Periodontists are skilled at removing teeth that are no longer viable due to dental or periodontal disease. If bone regeneration is needed in order to restore the removed tooth with a dental implant, the two procedures might be done in the same appointment.

- **Dental Crown Lengthening:** Some people with periodontal disease develop excess gum tissue. Other people naturally have a "gummy" smile. The dental crown lengthening procedure is used to surgically remove excess gum and bone tissue to expose more of the natural tooth. This can be done to one tooth or to several teeth prior to restoration with crowns and/or veneers. The results will be naturally beautiful teeth of even height and symmetrical gum contours framing the teeth. (See Figure B).

- **Dental Implants:** A dental implant is an artificial tooth root that is placed into the jawbone in order to hold a prosthetic tooth or bridge. The dental implants are tiny titanium posts that are surgically placed into the jawbone where teeth are missing. The bone bonds with the titanium, creating a strong foundation for artificial teeth. Small posts are then attached to the implant, which protrudes through the gums. These posts provide stable anchors for artificial replacement teeth. (See Figure C).

Dental implants can be used to support and retain full dentures for people who have lost their teeth and help preserve facial structure. Dental implant treatment is the gold standard of care today for the replacement of missing teeth due to its benefits. The benefits include elimination of further bone recession, stable prosthetic teeth that function like healthy natural teeth, ability to brush and floss easily, and longer lasting restorations.

The dental implant process is a team effort between a surgeon and a restorative dentist. While the periodontist performs the actual implant surgery, as well as the initial tooth extractions and bone grafting if necessary, the restorative dentist (your dentist) fits and makes the permanent prosthesis (artificial tooth). Your dentist will also make any temporary prosthesis needed during the implant process to replace any missing teeth. Dental implants give patients a permanent option for replacing missing teeth instead of using a bridge. Dental implants are comparable in cost to crown and bridge treatment. (See Figure D).

Figure A

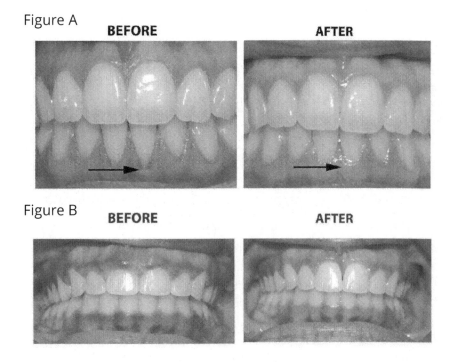

Figure B

Figure C

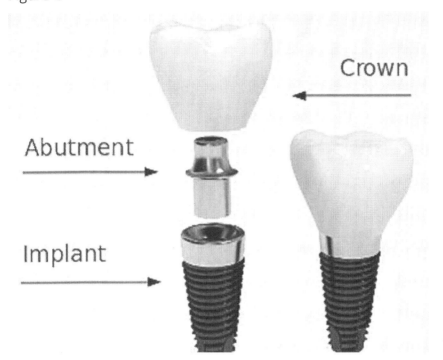

Crown

Abutment

Implant

Figure D

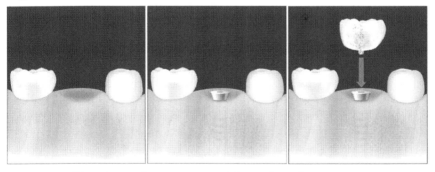

Tooth replacement with an implant

CHAPTER 3

YOUR ORAL HEALTH AND SPECIFIC SYSTEMIC DISEASES

The Diabetes Connection

Diabetes is a medical condition that arises when your blood sugar levels are higher than normal. There are two types of diabetes—type 1 and type 2. In the case of type 1 diabetes, your body does not produce insulin. In the case of type 2 diabetes, your body produces insulin but not in sufficient quantities.

Inflammation is a normal process that occurs as your body responds to germs or injury. Typical signs of inflammation can include an allergic reaction, swelling, redness in a wounded area, or a fever. While acute inflammation is necessary for your body to heal itself, inflammation that continues for a prolonged period (i.e., is chronic) results in adverse health conditions. Periodontitis is often stated to be the sixth complication of diabetes.

A 2001 study published in the journal *Annals of Periodontology* revealed a strong link between diabetes and periodontitis.[7] Many studies have followed. One hundred and fifty published studies demonstrating a clear two-way relationship between diabetes and periodontitis are presently listed in the US National Library of Medicine (National Institutes of Health). This means that if you have gum disease or periodontitis it can lead to diabetes and vice versa.

Inflammation Leads to Periodontitis and Diabetes

Periodontitis can change the action of insulin on glucose resulting in insulin resistance and high blood sugar. A 2005 study that investigated the link between diabetes, obesity and periodontitis revealed that having periodontitis can cause chronic inflammation in the body resulting in diabetes.[8] It is confirmed that periodontal disease is an aggravating factor among patients with diabetes and contributes to complications.

Medical researchers and physicians recommend that treating periodontitis and other minor gum diseases is crucial to prevent complications associated with diabetes. They also recommend healthy dietary and lifestyle changes. With appropriate food habits it is possible to lead a quality life that is free of other health complications. Preventive oral health measures should be taken such as regular teeth cleanings and checkups by your dentist and/ or periodontist.

Your Oral Health Can Influence Your Risk of Diabetes

According to a 2006 CDC report, diabetes affects nearly 20 million Americans, among which 35–40% of the cases remain undetected. The prevalence of diabetes for adults worldwide was estimated to be 6.4 percent in 2010 and is projected to be 7.7 percent in 2030. The total number of people with diabetes is projected to rise from 285 million in 2010 to 439 million in 2030. About 21 million Americans have diagnosed diabetes, almost 9 percent of the adult population, but diabetes rates are growing in the U.S. In fact, about 35 percent of Americans have pre–diabetes. African–Americans, Hispanics/ Latinos and other ethnic minorities bear a disproportionate burden of diabetes in the U.S.

How to Identify if You Have Diabetes

If you have type 2 diabetes the symptoms are mild and may often go unnoticed. Here are the common symptoms of diabetes.

- Excessive thirst

- Excessive urination

- Feeling tired

- Slow healing of cuts or wounds

- Dizziness

- Blurry vision

- Numbness in hands and feet

- Unexplained weight loss or gain

In order to determine if you have high blood sugar, your primary healthcare provider can order a fasting blood sugar test, glucose tolerance test, and random blood sugar analysis. Another efficient way to determine the blood sugar level is the A1C test.

Your body produces red blood cells that live for about three months. The **A1C blood test** (also known as the **hemoglobin A1C test**) measures the glucose that clings to red blood cells and thus is indicative of your average blood glucose for the last 2–3 months. The test result is reported as a percentage. The higher the percentage, the higher is your blood glucose level. A normal A1C value is less than 5.7%, as shown in the chart below. Since the A1C test gives your physician a good picture of your blood sugar control, it is the primary test for diabetes management.

Diagnosis*	A1C level
Normal	Below 5.7%
Diabetes	6.5% or more
Pre-diabetes	5.7% - 6.4%

Source: National Diabetes information clearinghouse (NDIC)

*Any test for the diagnosis of diabetes requires confirmation with a second measurement unless there are clear symptoms of diabetes. Since diabetes leads to other health complications with other body functions such as eyes, heart, kidneys, nerves and feet, it is important to take preventive measures in order to reduce the risk of diabetes. While there are many causes for diabetes, recent studies linking inflammation of the gums (gingivitis and periodontitis) to diabetes are cause for attentive oral hygiene, which include regular teeth cleaning and checkups by your dentist or periodontist.

Case Study One: Jim

Jim is a 45-year-old man who presented with an advanced case of periodontal disease. A 25-year smoker with a history of hypertension and diabetes, Jim rarely exercises, but attempts to control his conditions with medication and diet. Due to a lack of health insurance benefits, his dental visits over the years have been sporadic at best, which has led to a deterioration of his oral health. While he was aware of many of the risks associated with smoking, Jim did not know that it was also contributing to his periodontal condition. Despite the consequences, he still enjoys smoking and is not ready to give it up. Jim is advised to undergo periodontal treatment, not only to improve the health of his gums, but also to prevent his diabetes and hypertension from becoming worse.

According to the American Association of Periodontology, there is a strong link between gum disease and diabetes. It is therefore crucial that Jim and others with this disease seek regular periodontal assessments and treatment. Those with type 2 diabetes should be aware that, while basic periodontal care may not be enough to control glucose, advanced treatment can make a significant difference. Therefore, periodontal treatment will not only improve the conditions of Jim's gums, it also will improve his diabetic glucose and significantly reduce the bacterial load affecting his health.

Finally, Jim also has hypertension, which is a leading cause of heart attack and stroke. Since gum disease has been associated with cardiovascular disease, periodontal treatment will reduce Jim's risk of these life-threatening events.

The Connection Between Periodontitis, Metabolic Syndrome, and Obesity

Many individuals have Metabolic Syndrome (MS), also known as Reaven's syndrome, insulin resistance (IR) syndrome, plurimetabolic syndrome, and syndrome X. This syndrome is a characterized by multiple system abnormalities including hyperglycemia (high blood sugar), abdominal obesity, abnormal cholesterol and triglyceride levels, and hypertension. All of these abnormalities are also increased risk factors for periodontitis.

Obesity is an excess amount of body fat in proportion to lean body mass, to the extent that health is impaired. It is the most significant contributor to cardiovascular disease. The fatty tissue of obesity has been shown to function as endocrine organ which secretes numerous factors referred to as adipocytokines that can cause disease through dysregulated immune responses. Among those diseases are periodontitis, inflammatory bowel disease (IBD), and metabolic syndrome (MS).

Scientific data suggests that obesity and metabolic syndrome are precursors of type 2 diabetes mellitus. As previously discussed in this publication, multiple studies have shown a bi-directional relationship between periodontal status and diabetes. Researchers also have reported data that suggests the association between periodontitis and MS is bi-directional.[9] The continuous bacterial challenge of periodontitis leads to low grade chronic infection, which exacerbate the ongoing inflammation in distant organs. The immune system response to inflammation in organs, throughout the body, exacerbates the inflammation of periodontitis. Hence exists the hypothesis of bi-direction, and this hypothesis is the focus of many current studies.

Supporting this hypothesis is the two-way clinical observation of periodontal inflammation worsening when inflammatory markers associated with MS increase, and the clinical observation of the inflammatory components of MS increasing when periodontal inflammation persists.

Obesity, by itself and as a component of MS, can result in increased cytokines (chemical switches that turn certain immune cell types on and off), which, in turn, can worsen periodontitis and other inflammatory diseases of the body.[10-21]

Knowing that obesity is a growing national problem, in general, not for genetic reasons but because of dietary choices and sedentary lifestyle, dentists, periodontists, primary health care providers, and other health providers are alarmed and urging their patients to combat it. We have reached a point in the scientific evidence where the statistics cannot be denied. Both providers and the public are becoming super conscious of the connection between habitual healthy choices and systemic health. I predict we will be seeing a growing trend of health professionals, including dentists and dental specialists, branching out to provide more oral and systemic health risk assessment, nutritional consulting, and active lifestyle coaching as part of their practices.

The Cardiovascular Heart Disease Connection

Several studies have shown periodontal disease to be linked to arterial inflammation. [22] The American Heart Association, after reviewing numerous studies concluded there is "level A" evidence (superb studies in multiple populations) that periodontal disease is independently (after adjusting for a multitude of other known risk factors) associated with arterial disease. While a cause–and–effect relationship has not yet been proven, [23] researchers think that inflammation caused by periodontal disease is the most likely cause. Periodontal disease can exacerbate existing heart conditions. Patients at risk for infective endocarditis may require antibiotics prior to dental procedures. Your periodontist and cardiologist will be able to determine if this is necessary.

Additional studies indicate there is a relationship between periodontal disease and stroke. Studies have not only linked periodontal disease to Cardiovascular Heart Disease (CVD) and stroke, but they have also indicated dramatically increased risk of having CVD and/or stroke if periodontitis is present.[24] A 1999 study that adjusted for other risk factors demonstrated positive correlation between periodontitis and coronary heart disease.[25] In this 1999 study, those with extensive periodontal pockets had a C–reactive Protein (CRP) level 7 times higher, than those without periodontal disease. Their CRP levels were at levels significantly associated with risk of CVD and stroke. A 1993 study of 9,760 adults who were followed over a 14–year period found those who had periodontal disease were 25% more likely to develop coronary artery disease compared to those with minimal levels of periodontal disease. Males with periodontitis under the age of 50 were 72% more likely to develop coronary artery disease versus their counterparts.[26] A 1996 study reported a 50% increased risk of fatal CVD for patients age 30–40.[27] A 1997 study indicated a 250% increased risk of stroke.[28]

Note: Tobacco smoking and secondhand smoke increase the risk of CVD and other systemic diseases. Worldwide, tobacco smoking was one of the top three leading risk factors for disease and contributed to an estimated 6.2 million deaths in 2010. Sixteen percent of students grades 9–12 reported being current smokers. Among adults, 20 percent of men and 16 percent of women are smokers.

Statistics You Should Take to Heart

Cardiovascular Heart Disease (CVD) is the leading cause of death in the United States. An estimated 30 percent of deaths across the globe occur due to heart disease. According to the Global Burden of Disease Project, it is projected that by 2030, nearly 23.6 million people will die from heart disease and related conditions. Population studies and clinical research reveal that the majority of these deaths can be prevented by simple lifestyle changes like exercise and food habits.

According to the American Heart Association, six million CVD deaths are recorded globally per year. One-third of those are individuals less than 70 years old. Fifty percent of recurrent CVD events are fatal. Reported statistics underline the gravity of CVD:

Cardiovascular Disease Overall

- In 2008, cardiovascular deaths represented 30 percent of all global deaths, with 80 percent of those deaths taking place in low-income and middle-income countries.

- Nearly 787,000 people in the U.S. died from heart disease, stroke and other cardiovascular diseases in 2011. That's about one out of every three deaths in America.

- About 2,150 Americans die each day from these diseases, one every 40 seconds.

- Cardiovascular diseases claim more lives than all forms of cancer combined.

- About 85.6 million Americans are living with some form of cardiovascular disease or the after-effects of stroke.

- Direct and indirect costs of cardiovascular diseases and stroke total more than $320.1 billion. That includes health expenditures and lost productivity.

- Nearly half of all African-American adults have some form of cardiovascular disease—48 percent of women and 46 percent of men.

- Heart disease is the number one cause of death in the world and the leading cause of death in the United States, killing over 375,000 Americans a year.

- Heart disease is the number one killer of women, taking more lives than all forms of cancer combined.

- Over 39,000 African-Americans died from heart disease in 2011.

Cardiac Arrest

- In 2011, about 326,200 people experienced out-of-hospital cardiac arrests in the United States. Of those treated by emergency medical services, 10.6 percent survived. Of the 19,300 bystander-witnessed out-of-hospital cardiac arrests in 2011, 31.4 percent survived.

- Each year, about 209,000 people have a cardiac arrest while in the hospital.

Stroke

- Stroke is the number four cause of death in the United States, killing nearly 129,000 people a year.

- Someone in the U.S. has a stroke about once every 40 seconds. That is equivalent to 795,000 people every year.

- Stroke kills someone in the U.S. about once every four minutes. That's one in every 20 deaths per annum.

- Stroke is a leading cause of disability.

High Blood Pressure

- About 80 million U.S. adults have high blood pressure. That's about 33 percent. About 77 percent of those are using antihypertensive medication, but only 54 of those have their condition controlled.

- Nearly half of people with high blood pressure (46 percent) do not have it under control.

- Approximately 69 percent of people who have a first heart attack, 77 percent of people who have a first stroke and 74 percent who have congestive heart failure have blood pressure higher than 140/90 mm Hg.

- Hypertension is projected to increase about 8 percent between 2013 and 2030.

- Rates of high blood pressure among African-Americans are among the highest of any population in the world. Here is the U.S. breakdown by race and gender.

  - 46 percent of African-American women have high blood pressure.

  - 45 percent of African-American men have high blood pressure.

  - 33 percent of white men have high blood pressure.

  - 30 percent of white women have high blood pressure.

  - 30 percent of Hispanic men have high blood pressure.

  - 30 percent of Hispanic women have high blood pressure.

- In 2000, it was estimated that 972 million adults worldwide had hypertension.

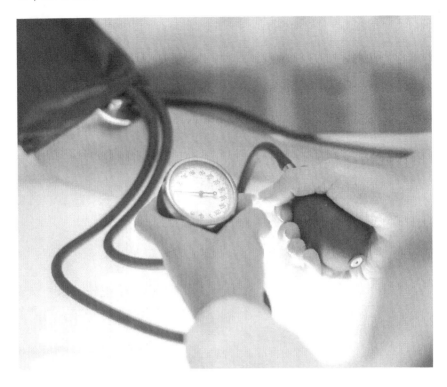

How to Help Prevent CVD and Stroke

Talk to your doctor and be aware of the risk factors that can lead to CVD and stroke. Be sure to take preventive measures that will reduce the risk, including changes in diet, cessation of smoking, regular exercise, weight control, regular medical exams, and compliance with prescribed medication for high blood pressure, as well as other cardiovascular conditions. Preventive measures most definitely include good oral hygiene at home, regular teeth cleaning, and check ups for periodontal disease. If gingivitis or periodontitis is present, do not delay treatment.

The Rheumatoid Arthritis Connection

Rheumatoid arthritis (RA) is an inflammatory condition that affects the joints in your body. The condition is characterized by painful and swollen joints with impaired ability to move. This systemic inflammation affects the synovial membrane (lining) of the joints and also affects other parts of your body. The condition is debilitating if left untreated and leads to severe damage to the joints resulting in permanent disability.

Although the cause of rheumatoid arthritis is not yet clear, researchers unanimously agree that inflammation is one of the primary factors that can trigger the disease. Recent findings indicate that gum disease (a primary source of inflammation in the body) can make your rheumatoid arthritis worse.

Researchers also have found that a particular gum bacterium called *Porphyromonas gingivalis* is present in the oral cavity, attacking your gum tissues as well as your jaw joints.[29] *Porphyromonas gingivalis* converts the arginine residues in protein molecules to citrulline. Citrulline is a protein that is present in the joints of patients suffering from rheumatoid arthritis. The conversion to citrulline is a step in the inflammatory process that leads to damage of the cartilage tissue and joints. This research made a strong connection between gum disease and rheumatoid arthritis.

How to Help Prevent Rheumatoid Arthritis?

Talk to your doctor and be aware of the risk factors that can lead to rheumatoid arthritis. Be sure to take preventive measures that will reduce the risk. Although the exact cause for rheumatoid arthritis is not clearly known, researchers strongly agree with the damaging role played by inflammation.

Case Study 2: Julie

Julie is a 39 year–old single mother and leukemia survivor. She had a rather difficult childhood and was determined to give her daughter a better life. When she came into the office for an exam, she was not aware of her periodontal condition; however, she had been noticing changes in her gums when brushing her teeth. During her pregnancy, Julie had experienced similar redness and puffiness of her gingival tissue. When she received professional care after giving birth, her condition improved, but a year later it had inexplicably worsened again. When her dentist noticed lesions on her gums, he referred Julie for a periodontal consultation.

During the assessment, it was revealed that Julie had been diagnosed with rheumatoid arthritis several years before. In fact she had recently been experiencing discomfort, not only in her back but in her jaw joints as well. It was explained to Julie that medical literature shows there is a strong link between periodontal diseases and rheumatoid arthritis. The culprit—the bacterium *Porphyromonas gingivalis*, causes gum disease and also accelerates the breakdown of bones and cartilage throughout the body. This would explain the pain Julie was experiencing in her jaws and back. Although she had always assumed that she had inherited "bad teeth" from her mother, she now understood the how her rheumatoid arthritis was a contributing factor in the continued deterioration of her periododontal condition and the importance of getting oral inflammation under control.

Note: Periodontal care is not something we usually associate with pregnancy; however, it has been shown that pregnant women with untreated gum diseases run a higher risk of delivering early and having a baby of low birth weight. Interestingly enough, pregnancy is also a risk factor for gum disease. To avoid this cycle, it is important for pregnant woman to get regular periodontal checkups as part of their prenatal care. While Julie was lucky to give birth to a healthy daughter despite her gum disease, it easily could have become a problem, especially given her other health conditions.

The Alzheimer's Disease Connection

Alzheimer's is a condition that slowly destroys brain cells leading to loss of memory and coordination. It is a progressive brain disease that is irreversible resulting in memory loss, poor thinking capabilities, and loss of ability to do simple tasks. It is not clear how Alzheimer's occurs, but experts believe that the process begins decades before the damage actually starts surfacing. A study reported at the first Alzheimer's Association International Conference on Prevention of

Dementia in 2005 and published in 2006, examined lifestyle factors of more than 100 pairs of identical twins.[30] All of the pairs included one twin who had developed dementia and one who had not. Because identical twins are genetically indistinguishable, the study involved only risk factors that could be modified to help protect against dementia. Twins who had severe periodontal disease before they were 35 years old had a fivefold increase in risk of developing Alzheimer's disease. Since this report, multiple studies have been done linking chronic inflammation such as periodontitis to tissue damage, including the brain. Among the most significant reports are two published within the last two years.

Dental researchers from the New York University analyzed 20 years of study data that link gum disease to Alzheimer's.[31] The analysis revealed that subjects with gum disease and no previous history of impaired brain function showed a higher risk of poor cognitive skills when compared to subjects without gum disease and no history of impaired brain function.

In other findings from the University of Central Lancashire, England, researchers identified gum disease causing bacteria in brain samples of patients with Alzheimer's. [32] According to the study, *Porphyromonas gingivalis* (gum disease–causing bacterium) were found in four out of ten samples of brain tissue from Alzheimer's patients. Researchers did not find the bacterium in the brain tissue samples of normal subjects of the same age group and concluded there is a strong association between gum disease and the risk of Alzheimer's.

The Respiratory Disease Connection

Research has shown that bacteria found in the oral cavity can be aspirated into the lungs to cause respiratory diseases such as pneumonia, especially in people with periodontal disease. Aspiration pneumonia is the second leading cause of death in nursing homes. A 2006 study provided evidence that improved oral hygiene and frequent professional oral health care reduces the progression or occurrence of respiratory diseases among high–risk elderly adults.[33]

The Osteoporosis Connection

Osteopenia is a reduction in bone mass due to an imbalance between bone resorption and formation, favoring resorption. This results in demineralization and eventually progresses into osteoporosis. Osteoporosis is a disease characterized by low bone mass. Individuals with osteoporosis have a high risk of bone fracture. Periodontitis is an inflammation of the supporting tissues of the teeth, resulting in resorption of the alveolar bone (jawbone), as well as loss of the soft tissue attachment that connects each tooth to the bone. Thus, periodontitis is a major cause of tooth loss in adults. Studies have associated patients with osteoporosis with greater severity of periodontitis.[34] If you have osteoporosis, beware that unrecognized gingivitis could flare into a severe inflammation. Be diligent with your regular dental exams and teeth cleanings, and comply with recommended treatment for any present periodontal disease.

Gum Disease and Women

A woman's periodontal health may be impacted by a variety of factors.

Puberty

During puberty, an increased level of sex hormones, such as progesterone and possibly estrogen, causes increased blood circulation to the gums. This may cause an increase in the gums' sensitivity and lead to a greater reaction to any irritation, including food particles and plaque. During this time, the gums may become swollen, turn red, and feel tender.

Menstruation

Occasionally, some women experience menstruation gingivitis. Women with this condition may experience bleeding gums, bright red and swollen gums, and sores on the inside of the cheek. Menstruation gingivitis typically occurs right before a woman's period and clears up once her period has started.

Pregnancy

Some studies have suggested the possibility of an additional risk factor in pregnancy— periodontal disease. Pregnant women who have periodontal disease may be more likely to have a baby that is born too early and too small. However, more research is needed to confirm how periodontal disease may affect pregnancy outcomes.

All infections are cause for concern among pregnant women because they pose a risk to the health of the baby. The American Academy of Periodontology now recommends that women considering pregnancy have a periodontal evaluation.

Link to Pre-Term Birth and Preeclampsia

Several studies suggest that periodontal disease may be a potential risk factor for preterm low birth weight babies.[35] A study reported in 2006 found an association between the presence of chronic periodontal disease and preeclampsia in pregnant women.[36] A total of 83 out of 130 preeclamptic women (63.8%) had chronic periodontitis, compared with 89 out of 243 controls (36.6%) who did not experience preeclampsia. Preeclampsia is a disorder that occurs during pregnancy and the postpartum period that affects at least 5–8% of all pregnancies, it is a rapidly progressive condition characterized by high blood pressure and the presence of protein in the urine. Proper prenatal care is essential to diagnose and manage preeclampsia. Globally, preeclampsia as well as other hypertensive disorders of pregnancy are a leading cause of maternal and infant illness and death. By conservative estimates, these disorders are responsible for 76,000 maternal and 500,000 infant deaths each year.

Since periodontitis and its causes may be associated risk factors for preterm babies and since the mortality of low birth weight babies is on the rise, pregnant women should be screened for their oral health condition, educated about the connection and promptly referred for oral health care.

Menopause and Post-Menopause

Women who are menopausal or postmenopausal may experience changes in their mouth. They may notice discomfort in the mouth, including dry mouth, pain and burning sensations in the gum tissue, and altered taste, especially salty, peppery, or sour.

In addition, menopausal gingivostomatitis affects a small percentage of women. Gums that look dry or shiny, bleed easily, and range from abnormally pale to deep red mark this condition. Most women find that estrogen supplements help to relieve these symptoms.

Link to Pancreatic, Kidney and Blood Cancers

Research has shown that men with a history of periodontal disease had a 14 percent higher risk of cancer than those who did not have periodontal disease.[37] While the overall risk was 14 percent, the risk for specific cancers was typically higher. Compared to men with healthy gums, men with a history of gum disease had a 36 percent increased risk of lung cancer, a 49 percent hike in risk of kidney cancer, a 54 percent higher risk of pancreatic cancer, and a 30 percent increased risk of white blood cell cancers.

Link to Human Papillomavirus (HPV) Related Head and Neck Cancers

The incidence of oral cavity cancers has been steadily rising in the United States since 1973, despite the significant decline in tobacco use. The same trend has been reported in other parts of the world as well. This is attributed to a rise in sexual transmission of the oral HPV infection. According to data published in the *Archives of Otolaryngology — Head & Neck Surgery in 2012,*[38] you may be at a higher risk for head and neck tumors positive for human papillomavirus (HPV) if you have a history of periodontitis. The researchers noted that periodontitis is easy to detect and may represent a clinical high-risk profile for oral HPV infection. Saliva DNA testing can determine if a patient's periodontitis involves the HPV gene. Regular oral cancer screenings are essential, and even more so if you have a history of periodontitis. Preventing and treating inflammation in the oral cavity could be a simple and effective way to prevent and reduce oral HPV infection.

The Obstructive Sleep Apnea Connection

Sleep apnea occurs when tissue in the back of the throat collapses and blocks the airway, reducing the amount of oxygen delivered to all of your organs including your heart and brain. People with sleep apnea may snore loudly and stop breathing for short periods of time. When the blood–oxygen level drops low enough, the body momentarily wakes up. It can happen so fast that you may not be aware you woke up. This can happen hundreds of times a night, and you may wake up in the morning feeling unrefreshed.

A 2013 report in the *Journal of Periodontal Research* described a study of 687 individuals, whereas 460 were men and 227 were women, 47–77 years of age.[39] Sixty percent of those diagnosed with periodontitis also had obstructive sleep apnea (OSA). Obstructive sleep apnea (OSA) is a common disorder that is characterized by repeated disruptions in breathing during sleep, and mouth breathing. According to the American Sleep Apnea Association, 22 million Americans suffer from this condition. Eighty percent of those cases go undiagnosed. In part, this is because most patients do not realize that their snoring could indicate a larger concern.

Some common signs of sleep apnea include: loud snoring, insomnia, waking from sleep with a choking sound or gasping for breath, unrefreshed sleep, general daytime sleepiness, unintentionally falling asleep during the day, and fatigue. If you have these symptoms, you might have sleep apnea. If you suffer from OSA, you have an increased risk for high blood pressure, heart attack, and stroke. OSA has also been linked to diabetes, obesity, and depression. Discuss snoring and OSA treatment with your primary physician, dentist, and/or periodontist.

Oral appliance therapy (OAT) is an effective treatment option for patients with mild to moderate obstructive sleep apnea (OSA).

Although continuous positive airway pressure (CPAP) therapy is the first line of treatment for sleep apnea, many patients prefer an oral appliance to CPAP. An oral appliance is a small plastic device that fits in the mouth like a sports mouth guard or orthodontic retainer. Oral appliances help prevent the collapse of the tongue and soft tissues in the back of the throat, keeping the airway open during sleep and promoting adequate air intake. Oral appliances may be used alone or in combination with other treatments for sleep–related breathing disorders, such as weight management, surgery or CPAP. If you have been diagnosed with OSA, do not put off having regular teeth cleaning and oral checkups to prevent and treat gum disease.

The Inflammatory Bowel Disease Connection

Inflammatory bowel disease (IBD) is a chronic inflammation of all or part of the digestive tract. Ulcerative colitis and Crohn's disease are two manifestations of IBD. Both usually involve severe diarrhea, pain, fatigue, and weight loss. Ulcerative colitis is a disease in the large intestine that causes inflammation and ulcers filled with pus and mucus. Crohn's disease can occur anywhere in the digestive tract and often spreads deep into the layers of affected bowel tissue. According to the Crohn's & Colitis Foundation of America (CCFA), research indicates that a combination of four factors leads to IBD: a genetic component, an environmental trigger, an imbalance of intestinal bacteria, and an inappropriate reaction from the immune system. Immune cells normally protect the body from infection, but in people with IBD, the immune system mistakes harmless substances in the intestine for foreign substances and launches an attack, resulting in inflammation.

The Importance of Diagnosis and Medical Management

Both ulcerative colitis and Crohn's disease can be painful and debilitating. Life threatening complications can occur, including deep ulcerations, bowel obstructions, infections and malnutrition. Patients with IBD are at an increased risk for colon cancer. They are also at risk of the liver becoming inflamed and damaged.

An often–confused complex of symptoms known as irritable bowel syndrome (IBS) is not an infection and does not cause ulcers or other damage to the bowel. The symptoms of IBS include crampy pain, bloating, gas, and mucus in the stool, diarrhea, and constipation. Although uncomfortable, IBS has not been associated with life threatening complications. Individuals with IBD can also experience all of the IBS symptoms.

Since IBD can progress in severity and suddenly become life threatening, accurate diagnosis and medical management by gastrointestinal specialists is important. The diagnosis of IBD can involve blood tests, stool tests, endoscopic imaging of the inside of the upper and lower digestive tract, and external CT or MRI imaging.

What We Know about the Link Between IBD and Periodontitis

The oral cavity is frequently affected in patients with inflammatory bowel disease (IBD), especially in patients with Crohn's disease (CD). In an 8–month study at the Laboratory for Immunohistochemistry and Immunopathology at the University of Oslo, Norway, systematic oral examinations were performed in 113 patients with IBD, including 69 patients with CD and 44 patients with ulcerative colitis. One hundred thirteen healthy volunteers served as a control group. IBD, and especially perianal disease in CD, was found to be associated with periodontitis. Researchers concluded that optimal therapeutic strategies should probably focus on treating both the local oral and systemic inflammation.[40] Both IBD and CD are thought to be caused by immunological hypersensitivity to gut bacteria. Local hypersensitivity to bacteria in the mouth likewise causes periodontal disease.[41] In both cases, Helicobacter pylori bacteria is characteristic of the mucosa inflammation. It is thought that this bacteria present in the oral cavity is a source of gastric infection.[42]

If you have IBD, frequent periodontal assessment, and care by your dentist or periodontist will reduce the bacteria that can trigger or exacerbate gastric infection. This will help improve your quality and longevity of life.

Gum Disease and Children

Types of Periodontal Diseases in Children

- Chronic gingivitis is common in children. It usually causes gum tissue to swell, turn red, and bleed easily. Gingivitis is both preventable and treatable with a regular routine of brushing, flossing, and professional dental care. However, left untreated, it can eventually advance to more serious forms of periodontal disease.

- Aggressive periodontitis can affect young people who are otherwise healthy. Localized aggressive periodontitis is found in teenagers and young adults and mainly affects the first molars and incisors. It is characterized by the severe loss of alveolar (jaw) bone, and ironically, patients generally form very little dental plaque or calculus (tartar).

- Generalized aggressive periodontitis may begin around puberty and involve the entire mouth. It is marked by inflammation of the gums and heavy accumulations of plaque and calculus. Eventually it can cause the teeth to become loose.

Importance of Good Dental Hygiene in Adolescents

Hormonal changes related to puberty can put teens at greater risk for getting periodontal disease. During puberty, an increased level of hormones, such as progesterone and possibly estrogen, cause increased blood circulation to the gums. This may cause an increase in the gums' sensitivity and lead to a greater reaction to any irritation, including food particles and plaque. During this time, the gums may become swollen, turn red, and feel tender.

As teen progresses through puberty, the tendency for the gums to swell in response to irritants will lessen. However, during puberty, it is very important to follow a good at-home dental hygiene regimen, including regular brushing and flossing, and regular dental care. In some cases, a dental professional may recommend periodontal therapy to help prevent damage to the tissues and bone surrounding the teeth.

Advice for Parents

Early diagnosis is important for successful treatment of periodontal diseases. Therefore, it is important that children receive a comprehensive periodontal examination as part of their routine dental visits. Be aware that if your child has an advanced form of periodontal disease, this may be an early sign of systemic disease. A general medical evaluation should be considered for children who exhibit severe periodontitis, especially if it appears resistant to therapy.

The most important preventive step against periodontal disease is to establish good oral health habits with your child. Here are basic preventive steps to help your child maintain good oral health:

1. Establish good dental hygiene habits early. When your child is 12 months old, you can begin using toothpaste when brushing his or her teeth. When the gaps between your child's teeth close, it's important to start flossing.
2. Serve as a good role model by practicing good dental hygiene habits yourself.
3. Schedule regular dental visits for family checkups, periodontal evaluations, and cleanings.
4. Check your child's mouth for the signs of periodontal disease, including bleeding gums, swollen and bright red gums, gums that are receding away from the teeth, and bad breath.

The progression of gum disease can be halted if the bacteria and debris are removed from the pockets in the gums. In years past, traditional gum treatment consisted of cutting away the diseased gum with the hope that the remaining tissue would heal and be healthy. Fortunately, a variety of new techniques have allowed us to treat chronic gum infections much more conservatively. Removing large amounts of diseased gum and then "packing" the gums is a thing of the past.

CHAPTER 4

YOUR MOUTH—YOUR RESPONSIBILITY

How is Your Oral Health?

Having read this book so far, you might be thinking, "Yikes! I wonder if I am at high risk for periodontal disease—and if I have it but don't know it."

Some Health Assessment Tools

Oral Health: To help you learn more about the state of your oral health, the American Academy of Periodontology has developed two online periodontal assessment tools. Feel free to print these from the Internet and share them with your dental professional. Ask your oral health provider any questions you have about your oral health. Please visit www.perio.org for the checklist and assessment test below.

Comprehensive Periodontal Evaluation Checklist

Gum Disease Risk Assessment Test

Diabetes: To help you learn about your risk for type 2 diabetes, the American Diabetes Association has developed an online Diabetes Risk Test. Complete the online test at www.diabetes.org and discuss the results with your primary and oral health care providers. If you are at high risk for diabetes, realize that any periodontal disease will heighten your risk.

Obstructive Sleep Apnea: Three tests that you can take right now to assess your risk for Obstructive Sleep Apnea (OSA) are available on the American Sleep Apnea Association (ASAA) website – www.sleepapnea.org. These tests are the ASAA Snore Score, the Epworth Sleepiness Scale, and the Berlin Sleep Questionnaire. You will be asked to enter your body-mass index. If you don't know what your BMI is, visit the National Heart Lung and Blood Institute website – www.nhlbi.gov – and search the term "BMI" to help you calculate your BMI.

Chronic Systemic Inflammation: In addition to puffy and bleeding gums, some symptoms of chronic inflammatory disease include ongoing irritating pain in the joints or muscles, asthma and allergies that are becoming worse, high blood pressure, blood sugar problems, ulcers, ongoing constipation or diarrhea, constant fatigue and skin problems. Discuss these symptoms with your doctor. Blood tests can be run to look for inflammatory markers. **Six common markers are:**

- **SED rate**—The sedimentation rate of erythrocyte is used in combination with other diagnostics to diagnose and monitor inflammatory disease.

- **Elevated high sensitivity C-reactive protein (HS-CRP)**—High levels of this protein are associated with cardiovascular disease.

- **Elevated homocysteine**—High levels of this amino acid are associated with cardiovascular disease.

- **Elevated ferritin (iron)**—High levels of iron can indicate the presence of a chronic disease process.

- **Elevated HDL**—High levels of "good cholesterol" can be indicative of a chronic inflammatory disease.

- **Elevated monocytes**—An increase in monocytes occurs as a response to chronic infection, autoimmune disorders, blood disorders, and cancer.

- **Elevated blood glucose**—High blood glucose happens when the body has too little insulin or when the body can't use insulin properly. Chronic occurrence is indicative of diabetes.

Simple Tips for Better Health Now

Everywhere we look, we are inundated with information about the importance of being healthy and how we can get healthy. Health is big business, with many experts claiming to know the "right" way to improve our health and the products we need in order to do so. Think about the TV commercials you see during the course of a day—they are pushing expensive workout equipment, diet plans that will deliver prepackaged foods to your home, and the latest new supplement that you *must* have in order to stay young and fit. In reality, it can be much simpler than that. While it is unfortunately more expensive to eat nutritious foods than it is to stop by the local McDonalds, there are choices each day that can improve your health without breaking the bank.

Similarly, improving your oral health does not have to be complicated; however, it does take diligence. You can prevent gum diseases by eating right and adopting certain preventive measures.

Periodontal Disease and Nutrition

Anti-oxidants and vitamins can play a role in fighting gum disease. In 2001, researchers at Loma Linda University reported the impact of an antioxidant-rich oral supplement on 63 patients ranging in age from 20 to 70 years, who had been diagnosed with gingivitis and Type II periodontal disease.[43] After 60 days, of a double-blind clinical trial, all subjects receiving the experimental treatment showed significant improvement. Several other studies have been done with anti-oxidants and vitamin B-complex, vitamin C, vitamin D, and dietary calcium. All of these studies suggested some therapeutic value when combined with conventional periodontal treatment. The current federal recommended daily allowance of vitamin D is 600 international units (IU) for adults up to age 70 (and 800 IU for those older than 70).

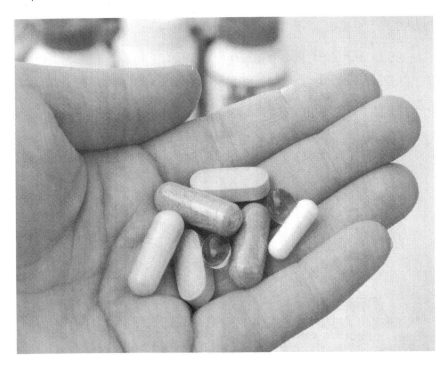

There are many studies linking free radical damage at the cellular level not only to premature aging, but also to virtually everything that ails us including periodontal disease. It is thought that safe nutritional supplements that neutralize the reactive oxygen species of bacteria in the periodontium can be of value in fighting periodontal disease, as well as all systemic inflammatory diseases.

It is generally accepted that daily nutrition with sufficient antioxidants, vitamin D, and calcium, will help prevent periodontal disease. A sufficient quantity of the vitamins is at the high end of their FDA recommended daily allowance. Your antioxidant levels can be raised by higher consumption of vegetables, berries and fruits or by phytonutrient supplements.

You are what you eat. Obesity has become an American epidemic, with nearly –seventy percent of adults being either overweight or obese. If you are one of them, your plan to become healthy must include a change in the way you eat. This means limiting certain carbs (those made with white flour, such as bagels and pasta), and eating more fish, fruits and vegetables. Particularly important for dental health is to cut down on sugary foods; however, this does not mean you need to deny yourself. When you are craving something sweet, reach for a low sugar granola bar, rather than a chocolate chip cookie.

Avoid processed foods: Processed foods are less nutritious and one of the primary reasons for dental caries because they are high in sugar. Sugar alters the salivary pH, composition of saliva, and also the integrity of the teeth making them more susceptible to plaque and dental caries.

Choose foods that are:

- **Rich in calcium and vitamin C:** Calcium rich foods like Kale, Brussels sprouts, sesame seeds, soybeans, mung beans, amaranth, and collard greens are safe and great sources of calcium. Vitamin C rich citrus fruits, kiwi, guava, and bell peppers are important for maintaining gum health. In addition, they also boost immune health and effectively fight infection.

- **Anti-inflammatory in nature:** Most plant-based foods are alkaline and promote anti-inflammatory effects in your body.

- **Herbs with anti-microbial properties:** Include herbs like parsley, coriander, cinnamon, spearmint, peppermint, rosemary, and tarragon. Their antimicrobial effects help to ward off bad breath and bad bacteria in the mouth. An additional bonus is that they aid in digestion, and some of them are also powerful antioxidants. Using toothpastes that contain these herbs or chewing on a teaspoon of the chopped herbs helps.

- **Take in more omega-3.** There has been promising research indicating that omega-3 fatty acids, found in salmon, mackerel and other fish, may help gum tissue heal. A recent Harvard Medical School study, which analyzed federal data tracking more than 9,000 people for five years, found that those who ate more fish rich in omega-3, or took a fish oil supplement, were up to 30 percent less likely to have gum disease.

Make Lifestyle Changes and Develop Healthy Habits

Stop smoking. Cigarettes and other tobacco products carry numerous health risks, including gum disease. It's no secret that quitting is extremely difficult for most people, so it's important to be systemic and organized. Find a smoking cessation program in your area for added support.

Get Moving. It is not necessary to join a gym or buy a treadmill to get fit. Find ways to incorporate physical activity into your daily life. Take the stairs instead of the elevator. Park at the far end of the parking lot, instead of right in front of the store. Take a walk before breakfast or after dinner. When you want to take it to the next level, get a jump rope and a pair of hand weights. You will feel better almost immediately, and it will make it much easier to lose weight.

Don't neglect your gums. Be sure to develop a routine for dental hygiene that includes brushing twice a day and flossing every day If possible, and make regular trips to the dentist. You should also have your gums checked each year, more often if you have a family history of periodontal disease, or other health conditions such as diabetes or heart disease.

Spend as much time as possible with people who share your health goals. If you are trying to quit smoking, it may be a while before you have the willpower to hang around people who are still puffing away. The same goes with food. It will require strength and commitment to resist the desserts your friends always put out, but one alternative is to invite them for a vigorous walk.

Find time to relax. Not only does stress erode our physical health, but it also causes us to revert to old, unhealthy coping mechanisms such as smoking and overeating. Now is the time to develop new ways to calm down. Take some time each day to unplug and do nothing. If you don't have a lot of time, start out with five minutes to just be quiet with yourself. Simply close your eyes, and take a few deep breaths. It helps to think of something—no matter how small—that you are grateful for. Also, be sure to get enough sleep each night.

Proper care and precautionary measures can prevent periodontal disease and also improve your overall health. Numerous patients coming through my practice have turned their oral health around, and in doing, so reduced the impact of systemic inflammatory disease. The following two case studies are examples.

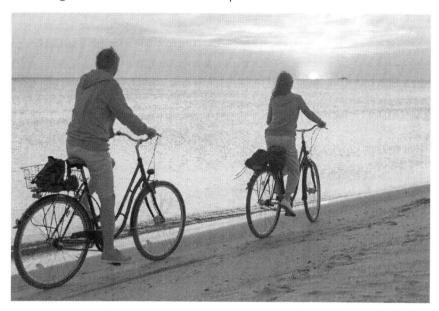

Case Study 3: George

George is a 64-year-old retired plumber raised on a farm. He grew up seeing his grandparents and parents wear dentures and believed it was inevitable that he would one day wear them as well. It's not that George doesn't want to keep his teeth; however, after several visits to the dentist where he heard things like "rampant caries" (widespread, rapidly progressing cavities), "periodontal disease" and "root decay," he had given up. He lost several teeth over the years and eventually had to have the remaining ones extracted. He was fitted for a removable denture, but unfortunately it is ill-fitting, uncomfortable, and moves whenever he tries to speak or eat.

George wants to regain a quality of life that includes enjoying the foods he loves and being able to speak clearly. If he continues to wear his dentures, they will continue to rock and slip, and his alveolar bone will continue to resors with the impact. This will not only affect the stability of his dentures, but also the amount of bone on which to place dental implants in the future.

While his situation may seem dire, George actually has several treatment options from which to choose. He can elect to have only two or three dental implants in the lower jaw to stabilize his current denture. Alternatively, he can also have four or five dental implants placed in the lower jaw, or six to eight in the upper jaw to have fixed restorations. Once he is healed, George's quality of life will drastically improve. He will have a natural smile, clear speech, and the ability to eat the foods he has been missing.

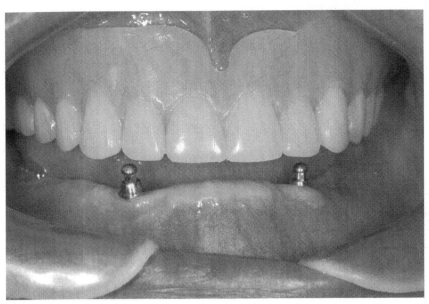

Case Study 4: Mary

Mary is a 57-year-old mother of five grown children and a grandmother of nine. After a lifetime of taking care of everyone else, Mary finally realized it was time to start taking care of herself.

Like most people, Mary has been through some struggles over the years, and the stress coupled with some unhealthy coping methods has taken its toll on her well being. She has been a heavy smoker for the past 45 years, which has had some devastating effects on her body. She suffered a heart attack, after which, a stent was placed in her heart. She is also battling osteoporosis and periodontal disease. Nevertheless, Mary is radiant, strong, and persistent—she is a fighter.

Unfortunately, by the time Mary sought periodontal treatment, her condition was rather advanced. It was too late to save most of her teeth, and those that were salvageable would not be strong enough to withstand the added pressure from a partial denture. Given the amount of bone loss, dental implants would be ideal; however, due to Mary's limited budget, they were not possible at this time.

This was disheartening for Mary, as she desperately wanted to be healthy and enjoy a renewed quality of life. Our recommended treatment plan was to remove the teeth that were hopeless, treat the remaining teeth with laser periodontal therapy, and provide upper and lower partial dentures in order to transition her into dental implants once her financial position improves.

After educating Mary on the devastating effects of periodontal disease in accordance with her overall health, Mary decided to move forward with the recommended treatment. She recovered better than expected, and, as a second oral DNA test confirmed, her bacterial load is significantly lower. With her periodontal status now stable, Mary has made a renewed commitment to her health. She has decided to quit smoking and has even joined a coaching program to help her achieve optimal overall health. As a result of these lifestyle changes, Mary is now enjoying a much greater quality of life and can expect to live longer. Her children and grandchildren look forward to having her around for a long time to come.

Final Words

Assess your risks for periodontal disease using the online tools recommended in this booklet. Realize that if you have systemic health issues, it is likely that periodontal disease is linked to these issues in some way through the inflammatory response system.

Although there are many things your dentist, hygienist and periodontist can do to help your mouth stay healthy, as well as restore a mouth ravaged by periodontal disease, you have the major responsibility for taking care of your teeth and gums. This includes proper nutrition, staying physically active, not smoking, brushing and flossing regularly, and having regular teeth cleanings and checkups. You are responsible for scheduling an annual physical exam so your primary physician can diagnose systemic diseases early. You are responsible for choosing to accept recommended treatment and for complying with healthcare provider instructions.

You will improve your overall health and the results of medical and dental treatment if you take the steps discussed in this booklet to eliminate and prevent periodontal disease. If periodontal disease is allowed to progress in your mouth, it is likely you will loose teeth. Do not allow it to progress. Reach out for help.

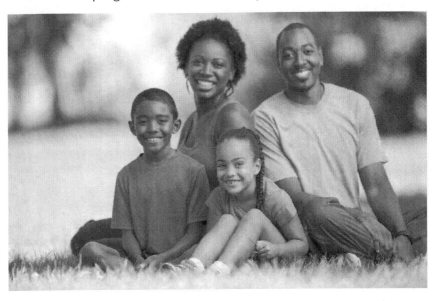

More Resources

For more resources to help you discover your oral and systemic health risks, please visit:

http://selfscreen.net/

http://selfscreen.net/21

BIBLIOGRAPHY

1. Pia, GW. Oral health and nutrition. Primary Care, 1994(1):121–33.

2. Ritchie, Christine, et al. Nutrition, inflammation, and periodontal disease. Nutrition and Oral Health, 2003(19):475–76.

3. Munoz C, Kiger R, Stephens J, Kim J, Wilson A. Effects of a nutritional supplement on periodontal status. Compendium, May 2001:425–38.

4. American Dental Hygienists' Association (ADHA) Fact Sheet .https://www.adha.org/resources-docs/7228_Oral_Health_Total.pdf

5. Rath SK et. Al. Periodontal pathogens in atheromatous plaque. Indian J Pathol Microbiol, 2014;57(2):259–64.

6. Preshaw PM, Bissett SM. Periodontitis: oral complication of diabetes. Endocrinol Metab Clin North Am, 2013;42(4):849–67.

7. Taylor GW, Bidirectional interrelationships between diabetes and periodontal diseases: an epidemiologic perspective. Annal Periodontol, 2001;6(1):99–112.

8. Pihlstrom BL, Michalowicz BS, Johnson NW. Periodontist and diabetes: a two-way relationshio. Lancet, 2005(366):1809–1820.

9. Han DH, Lim SY, Sun BC, Paek D, Kim HD. The association of metabolic syndrome with periodontal disease is confounded by age and smoking in a Korean population: The Shiwha–Banwol Environmental Health Study. J Clin Periodontol, 2010(37):609–16.

10. Jagannathachary S and Kamaraj D. J Obesity and periodontal disease. Indian Soc Periodontol. 2010;14(2):96–100.

11. Aronne LJ, Segal KR. Adiposity and fat distribution outcome measures: Assessment and clinical implications. Obes Res. 2002;10(Suppl 1):14S–21.

12. Lehr S, Hartwig S, Sell H. Adipokines: A treasure trove for the discovery of biomarkers for metabolic disorders. Proteomics Clin Appl. 2012(6)91–101.

13. Frayn KN, Williams CM, Arner P. Are increased plasma non-esterified fatty acid concentrations a risk marker for coronary heart disease and other chronic diseases? Clin Sci (Lond), 1996(90):243–53.

14. Saito T, Shimazaki Y, Koga T, Tsuzuki M, Ohshima A. Relationship between upper body obesity and periodontitis. J Dent Res. 2001(80)1631–6.

15. Saito T, Shimazaki Y, Kiyohara Y, Kato I, Kubo M, Iida M, et al. Relationship between obesity, glucose tolerance, and periodontal disease in Japanese women: The Hisayama study. J Periodontal Res. 2005(40):346–53.

16. Al-Zahrani MS, Bissada NF, Borawskit EA. Obesity and periodontal disease in young, middle-aged, and older adults. J Periodontol. 2003(74)610–5.

17. Wood N, Johnson RB, Streckfus CF. Comparison of body composition and periodontal disease using nutritional assessment techniques: Third National Health and Nutrition Examination Survey (NHANES III)J Clin Periodontol. 2003(30)321–7.

18. Linden G, Patterson C, Evans A, Kee F. Obesity and periodontitis in 60–70–year–old men. J Clin Periodontol. 2007(34)461–6.

19. Sarlati F, Akhondi N, Ettehad T, Neyestani T, Kamali Z. Relationship between obesity and periodontal status in a sample of young Iranian adults. Int Dent J. 2008(58)36–40.

20. Khader YS, Bawadi HA, Haroun TF, Alomari M, Tayyem RF. The association between periodontal disease and obesity among adults in Jordan. J Clin Periodontol. 2009(36)18–24.

21. Chaffee BW, Weston SJ. Association between chronic periodontal disease and obesity: A systematic review and meta–analysis. J Periodontol. 2010(81):1708–24.

22. Fifer KM, Qadir S, et al. Positron emission tomography measurement of periodontal 18F–Fluorodeoxyglucose uptake is associated with histologically determined carotid plaque inflammation. J Am Coll Cardiology, 2011(57):971–6.

23. Lockhart PB, Bolger AF, et al. Periodontal disease and atherosclerotic vascular disease: does the evidence support an independent association?: a scientific statement from the American Heart Association. Circulation, 2012(125)2520–44.

24. Beck J, Garcia R, Heiss G, Vokonas PS, Offenbacher S. Periodontal disease and cardiovascular disease. J Periodontol. 1996(67):1123–37.

25. Genco RJ, Wu TJ, Grossi S. Periodontal microflora related to the risk for myocardial infarction:a case control study. J Dent Res 1999;78:457.

26. DeStefano F, et al. Dental disease and risk of coronary heart disease and mortality. Br Med J 1993;306:688–691.

27. Beck J, et al. Periodontal disease and cardiovascular disease. J Periodontol, 1996(67: Suppl 10):1123–1137.

28. Grau AJ, Buggle F, et al. Association between acute cerebrovascular ischemia and chronic and recurrent infection. Stroke. 1997(28): 1724–9.

29. Pathirana RD, Neil M, et al. Host immune responses to Porphyromonas gingivalis antigens. Periodontology 2000. 2010(52):218–37.

30. Gatz M, Mortimer JA, et al. Potentially modifiable risk factors for dementia in identical twins. Alzeimer's & Dementia, 2006;2(2):110–7.

31. Kamer A, Pirraglia R., et al. Periodontal disease associates with higher brain amyloid load in normal ederly. Neurobiology of Aging. 2014. 36(2):627–33.

32. Poole S, Singhrao, SK, et al. Determining the presence of periodontopathic virulence factors in short–term postmortem Alzheimer's disease brain tissue. Journal of Alzheimer's Disease. 2013.

33. Azarpazhoo A, Leake JA. Systemic review of association between repiratory diseases and oral health. J Periodontol. 2006; 77(9): 1465-1482.

34. Esfahanian V, Mehrnaz S, et al. Relationship between osteoporosis and periodontal disease: review of the literature. J Dent (Tehran), 2010;9(4):256-64.

35. Shanthi V, Vanka A, et al. Association of pregnant women periodontal status to preterm and low–birth weight babies: A systemic and evidence–based review. Dent Res J. 2012;9(4):368-380.

36. Contreras A, Herrera JA, et al. Periodontitis is associated with preeclampsia in pregnant women. J Periodontol. 2006. 77(2): 182-188.

37. Michaud DS, et al. A prospective study of periodontal disease and pancreatic cancer in US male health professionals. J. Natl Cancer Inst. 2007(99):171-5.

38. Tezel M, Scannapieco FA, et al. Local inflammation and human papillomavirus status of head and neck cancers. JAMA, 2012;138(7).

39. Seo WH, Cho ER, et al. The association between periodontitis and obstructive sleep apnea: a preliminary study. J Periodontal Res. 2013;48(4):500-6.

40. Varicka SR, Manser CN, et al. Periodontitis and gingivitis in inflammatory bowel disease: a case–control study. Imflamm Bowel Dis. 2013;19(13):2768-77.

41. Brandtzaeg P. Inflammatory bowel disease: clinics and pathology. Do inflammatory bowel disease and periodontal disease have similar immunopathogeneses? 2001;59(4):235-243.

42. Namiot DB, Leszczynska K, et al. The occurrence of Helicobacter pylori antigens in dental plaque; an association with oral health status and oral hygiene practices. Adv Med Sci. 2010;55(2):167-71.

43. Munoz C, Kiger R, et al. Effects of a nutritional supplement on periodontal *status*. Compendium, May 2001:425-438.